E $10.95
Po   Poulet, Virginia
              Blue Bug's safety
           book

DATE DUE

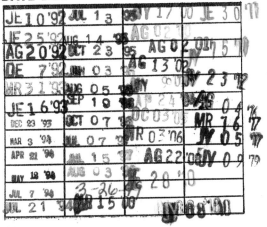

JE 10 '92	JUL 13	JY 17	JE 30
JE 25 '92	UG 14	AG 02	
AG 20 '92	OCT 23 '95	AG 02	5
DE 7 '92	JN 03	AG 13 '02	
MR 31 '9	UG 05	JY	JY 23
JE 16 '93	SEP 10	AP 24	AG 04
DEC 23 '93	OCT 07	OC 03 05	MR 16
MAR 3 '94	JL 07 '9	MR 03 '06	JV 05
APR 21 '94	JL 15	AG 22 '06	JV 09 '79
MAY 18 '94	AUG 03	2 0 '10	
JUL 7 '94	3-26-		
JUL 21 '94	JN 15 '00	JY 08 '00	

NO 2 4 '17

DEMCO

BLUE BUG'S
SAFETY BOOK

By Virginia Poulet
Illustrated by Donald Charles

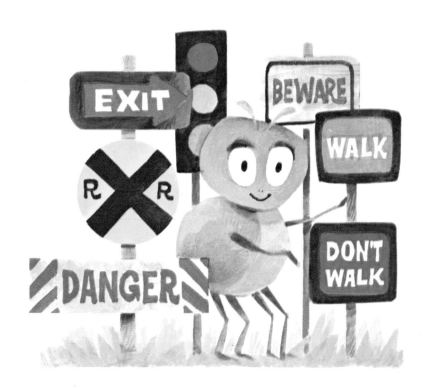

 CHILDRENS PRESS, CHICAGO

Library of Congress Cataloging in Publication Data

Poulet, Virginia.
  Blue bug's safety book.

  SUMMARY: By observing the safety signs, Blue Bug
arrives home unharmed.
  [1. Accidents—Prevention—Fiction] I. Charles,
Donald, illus. II. Title.
PZ10.3.P484Bn   [E]   72-8348
ISBN 0-516-03419-7

24 25 26 27 28 29 R 93 92 91 90

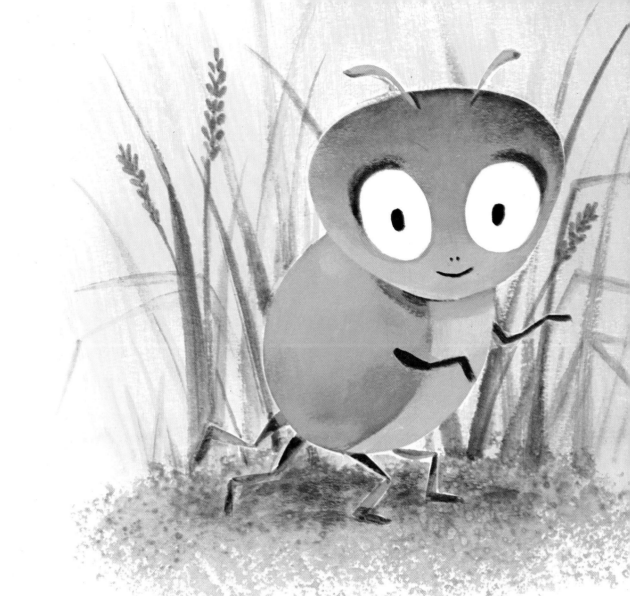

When
　　Blue Bug
　　　　walks home . . .

he must stop

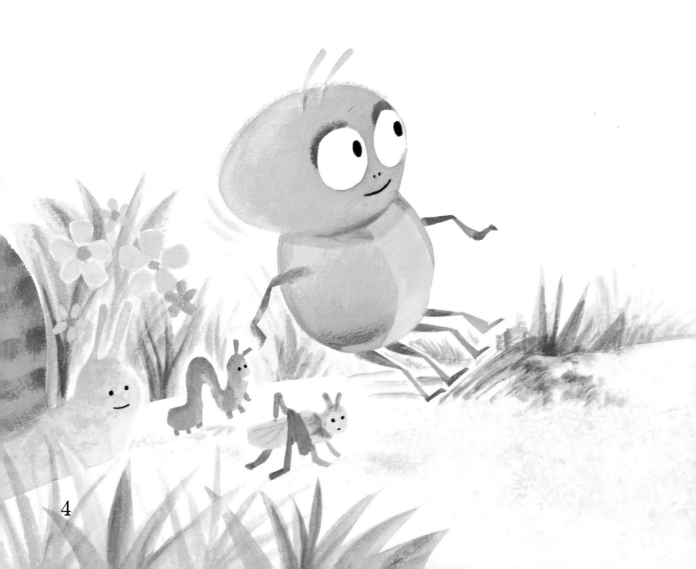

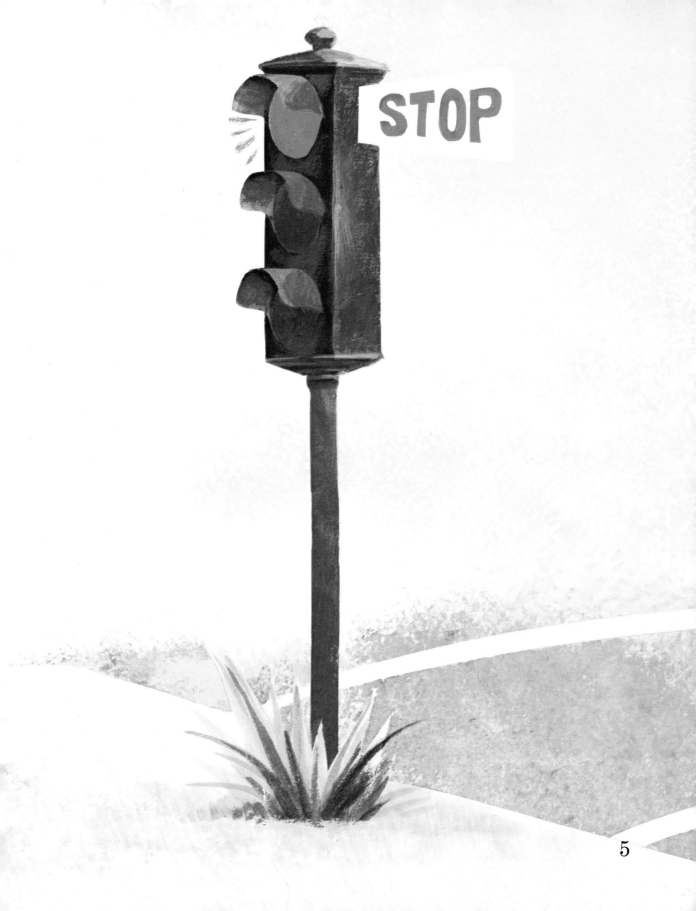

STOP

5

look

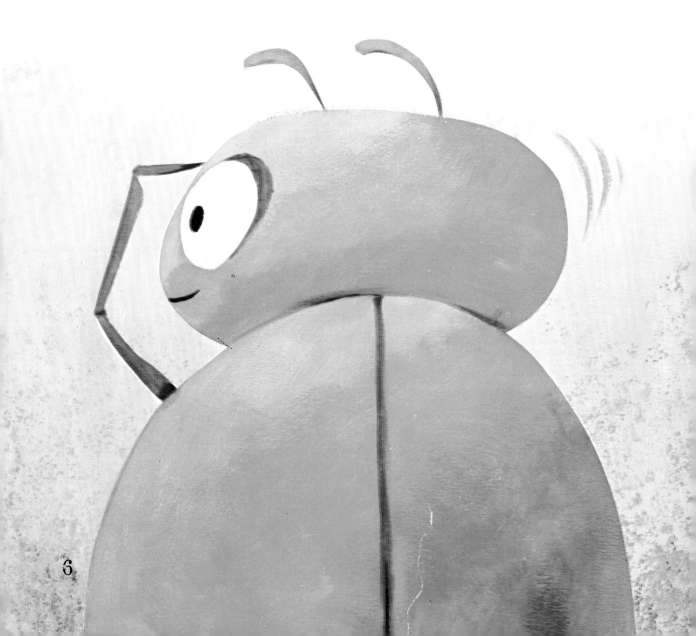

both ways

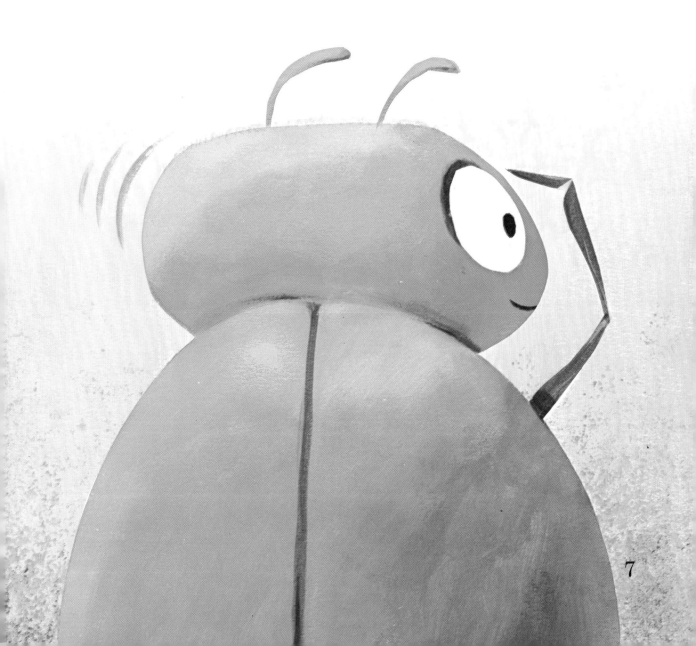

7

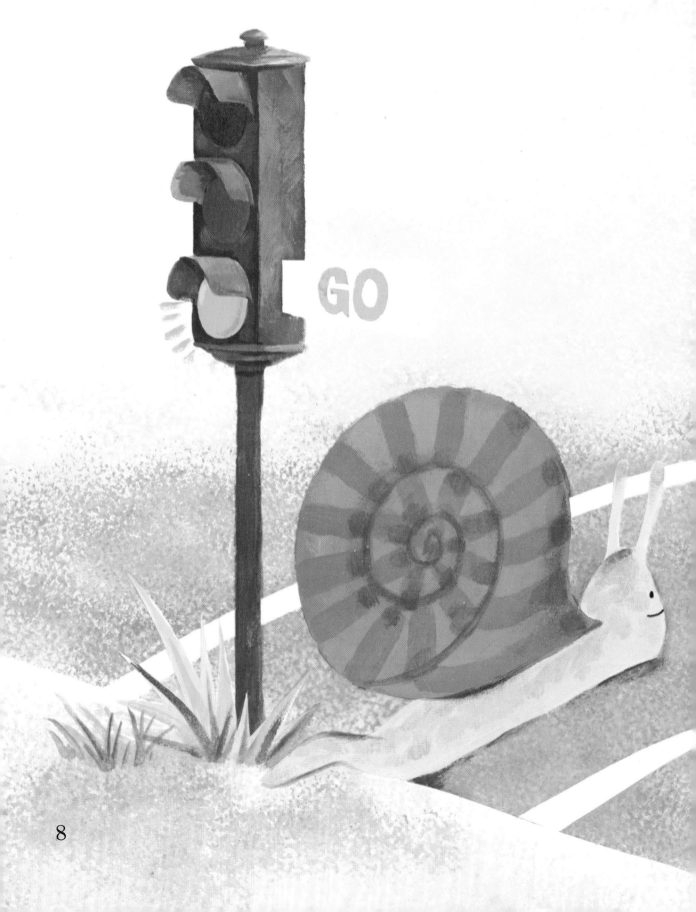

GO

8

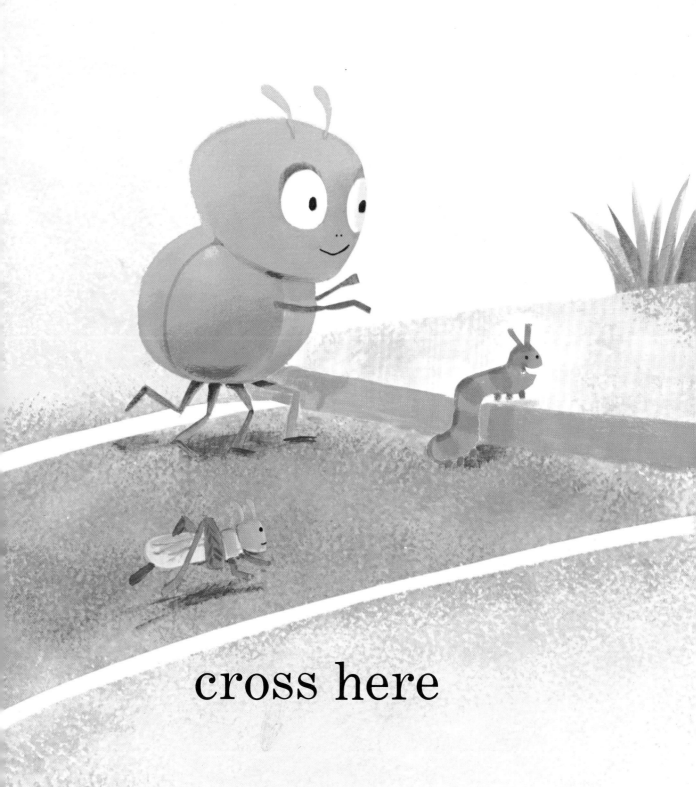

cross here

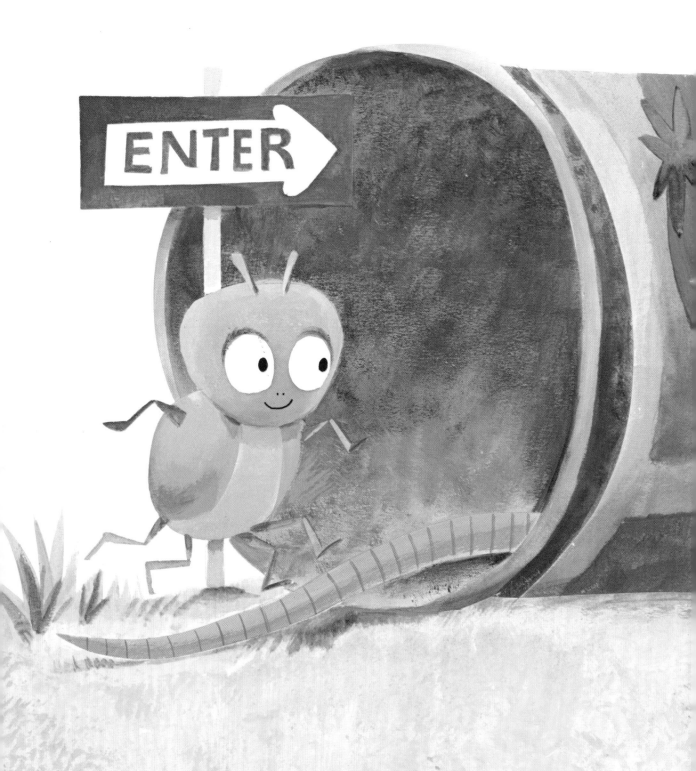

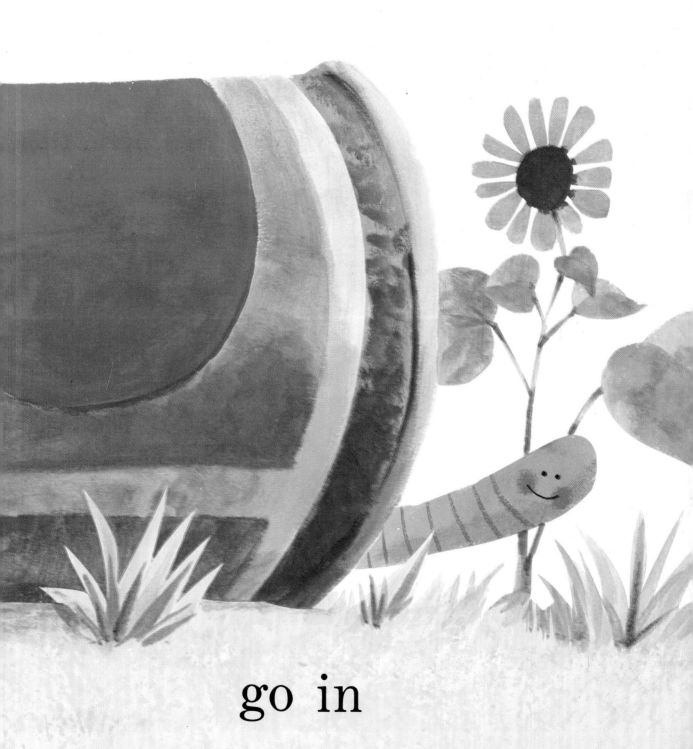

go in

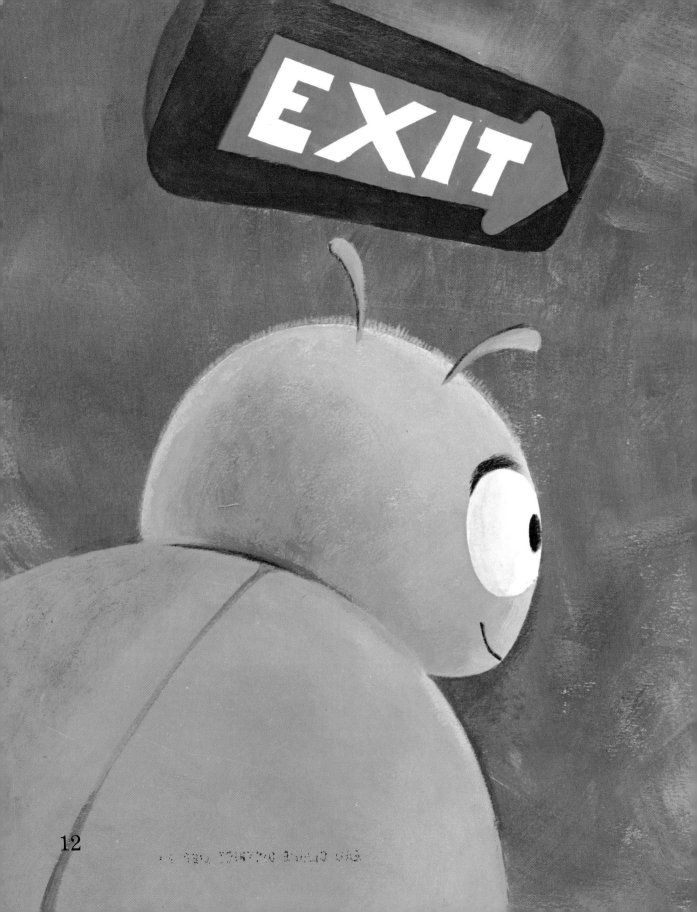

go out

13

watch his step

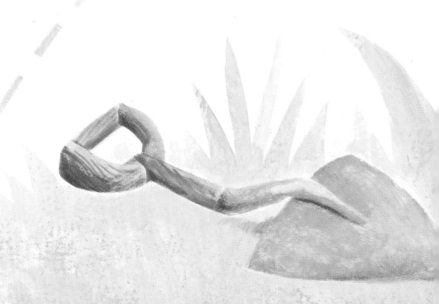

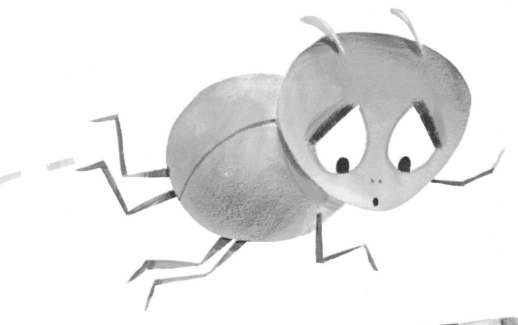

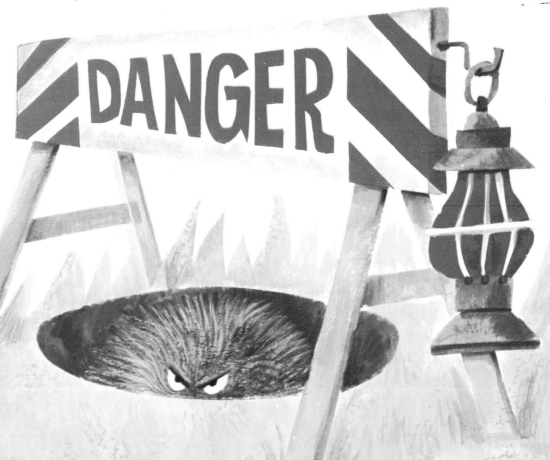

15

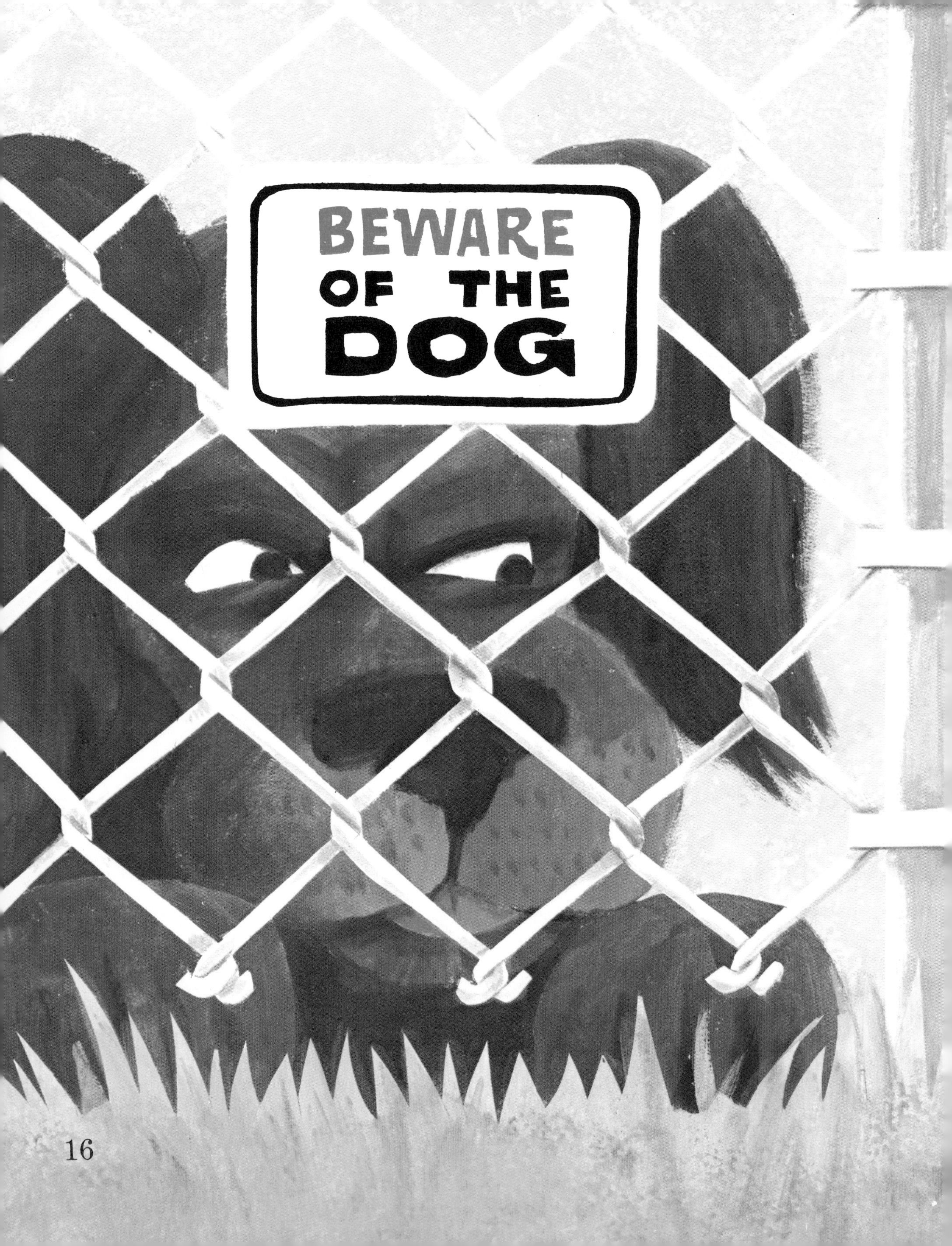
BEWARE
OF THE
DOG

be careful

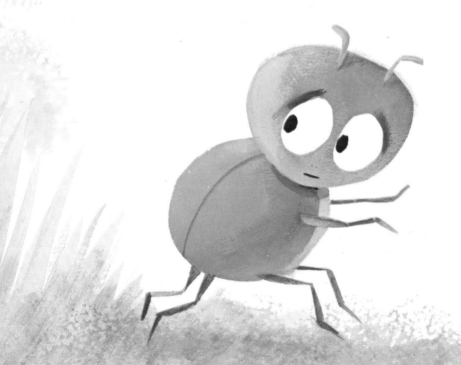

watch for trains

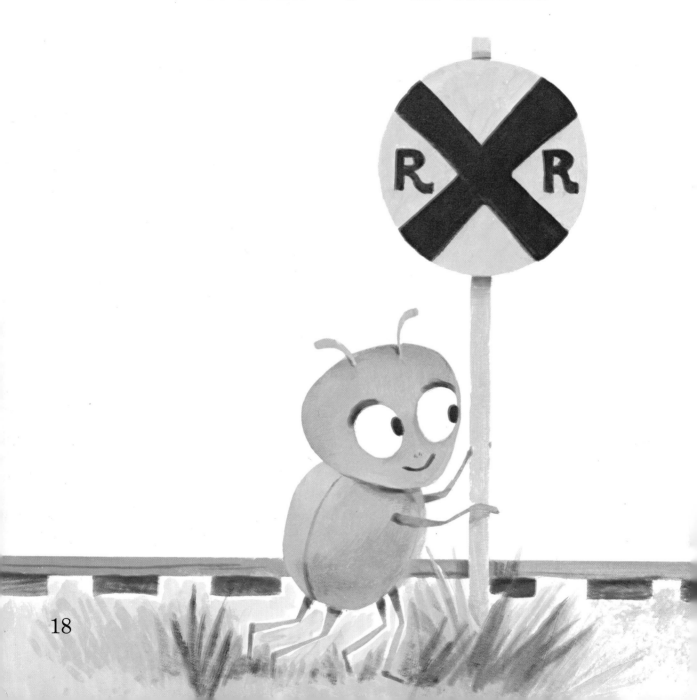

18

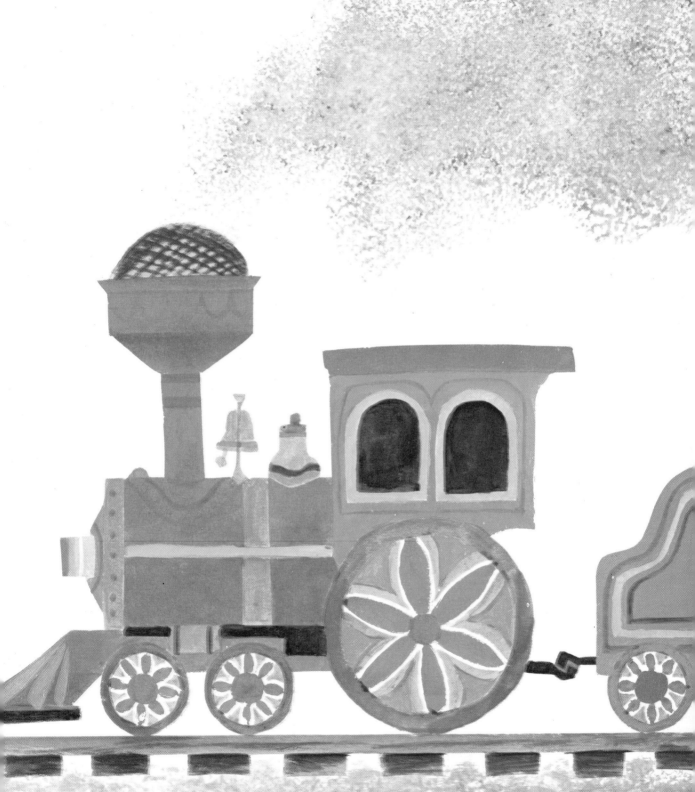

keep out

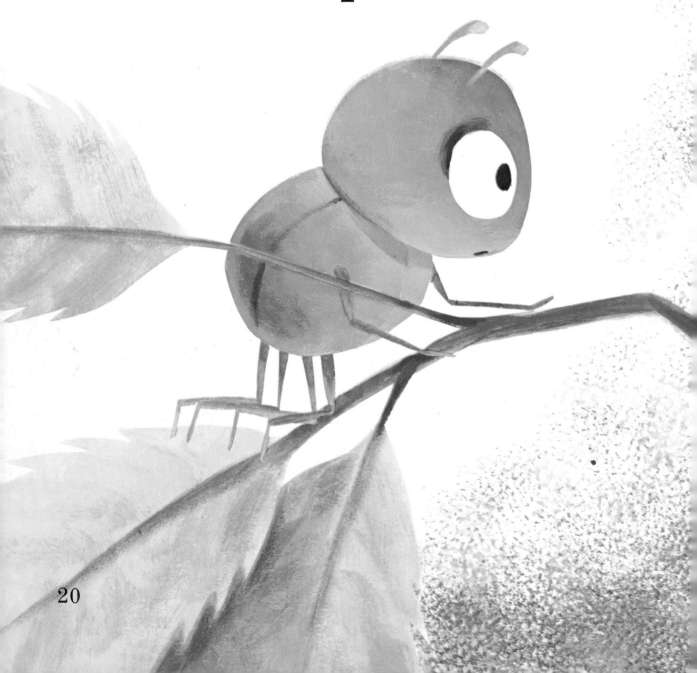

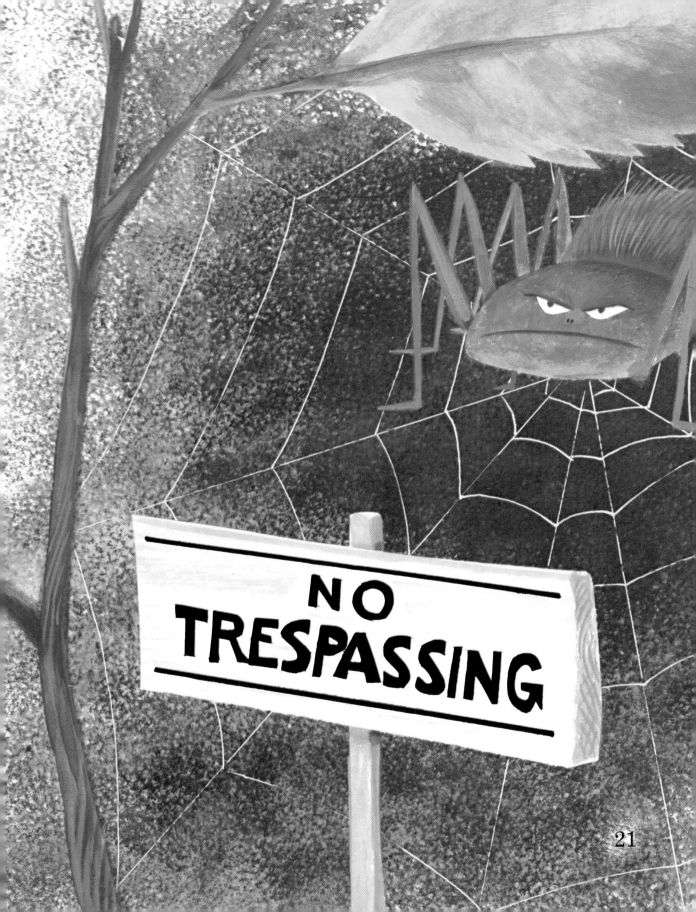

21

stay away

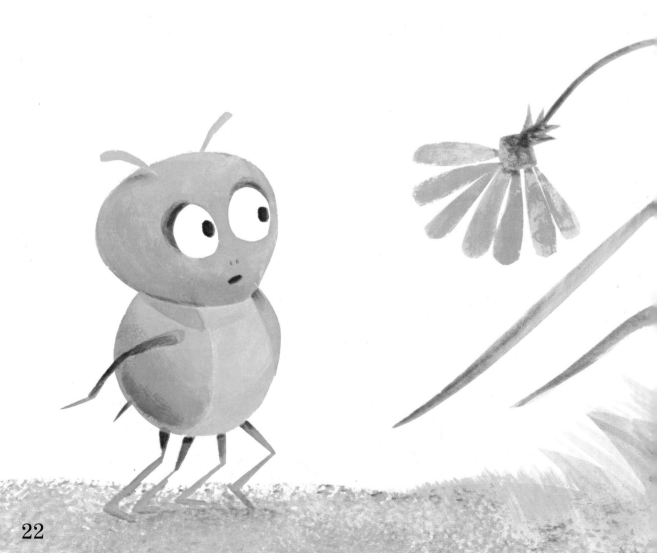

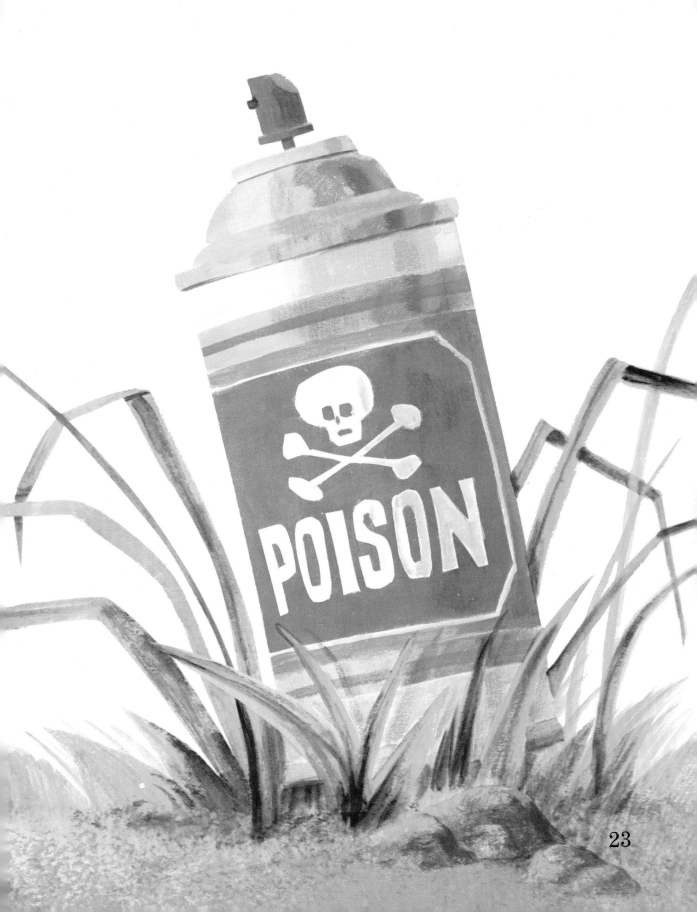

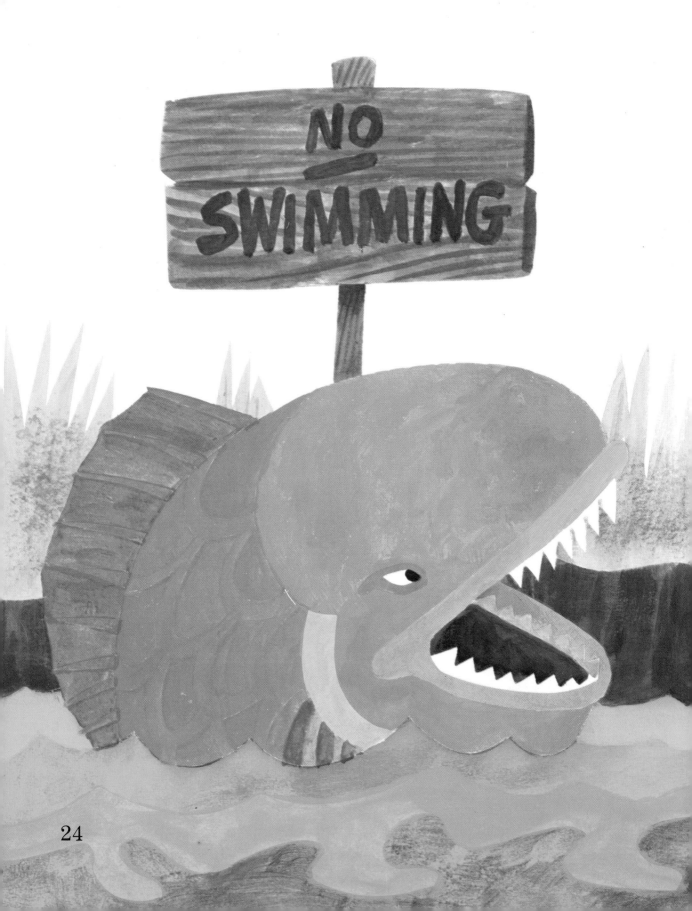

24

stay out

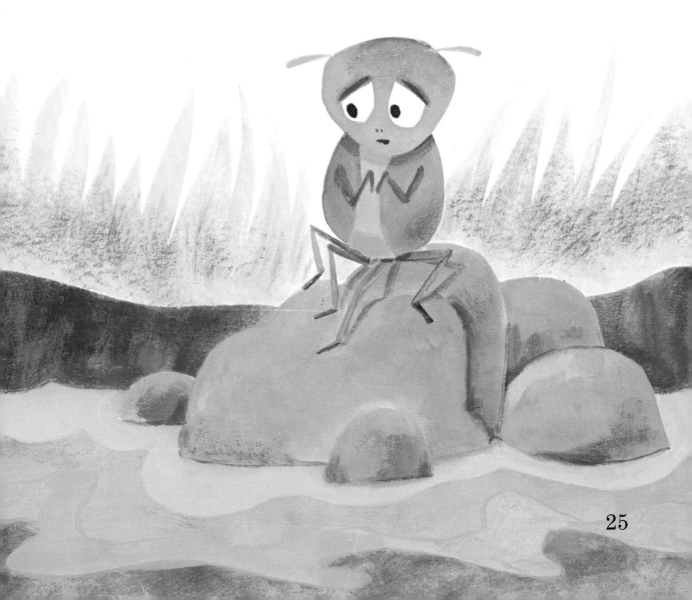

wait

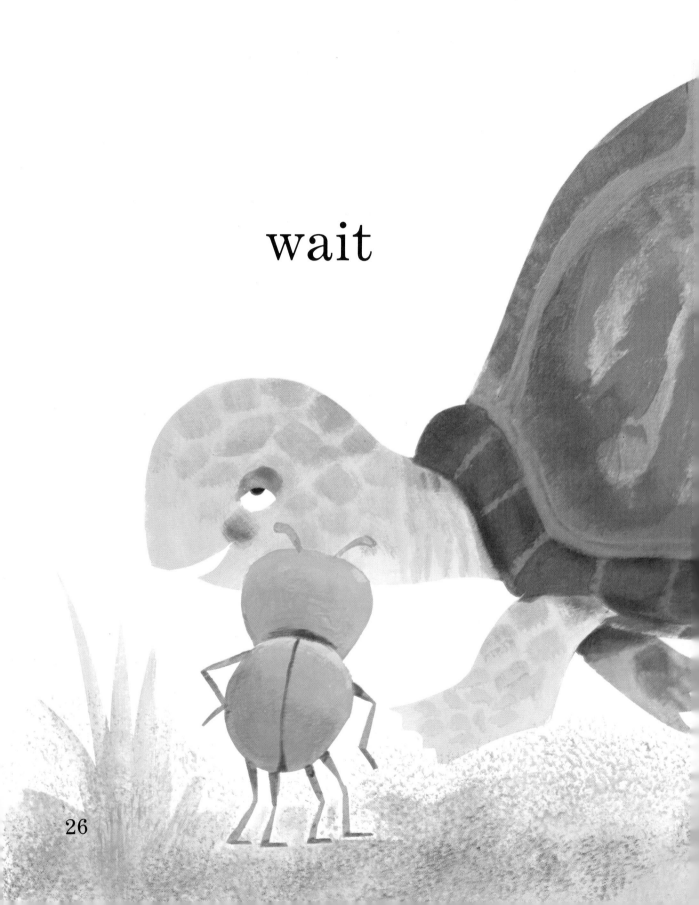

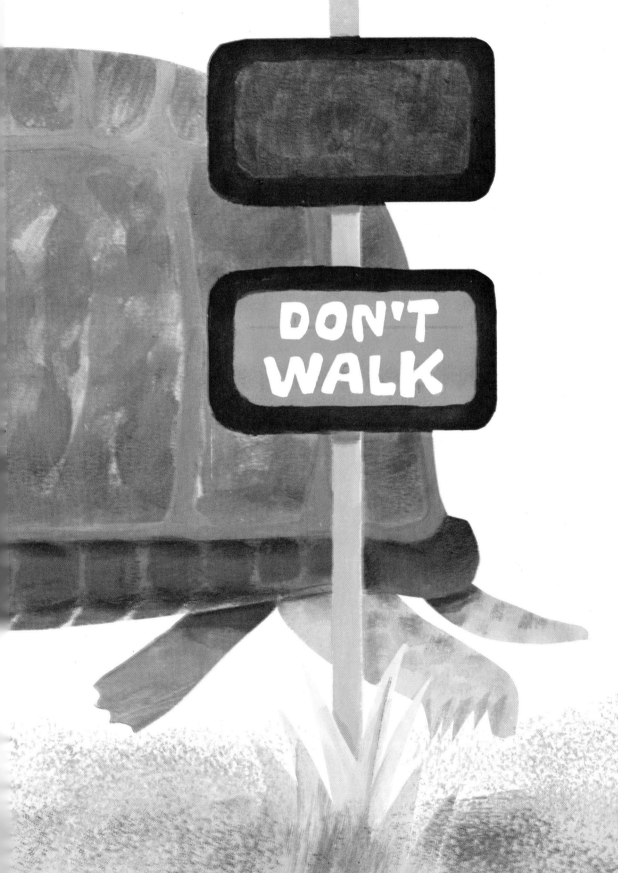

go.

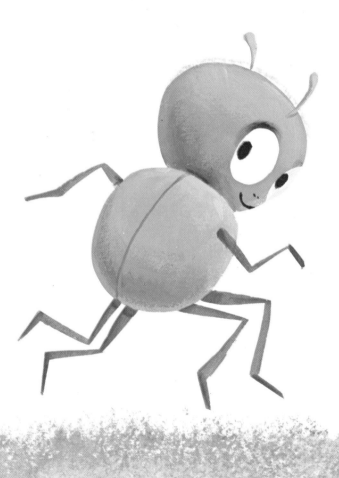

Blue Bug got home safely. He knows the safety signs.

Do you?

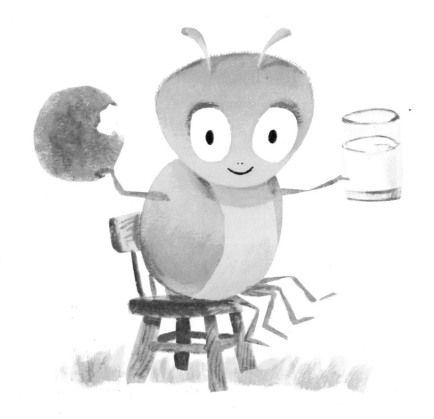

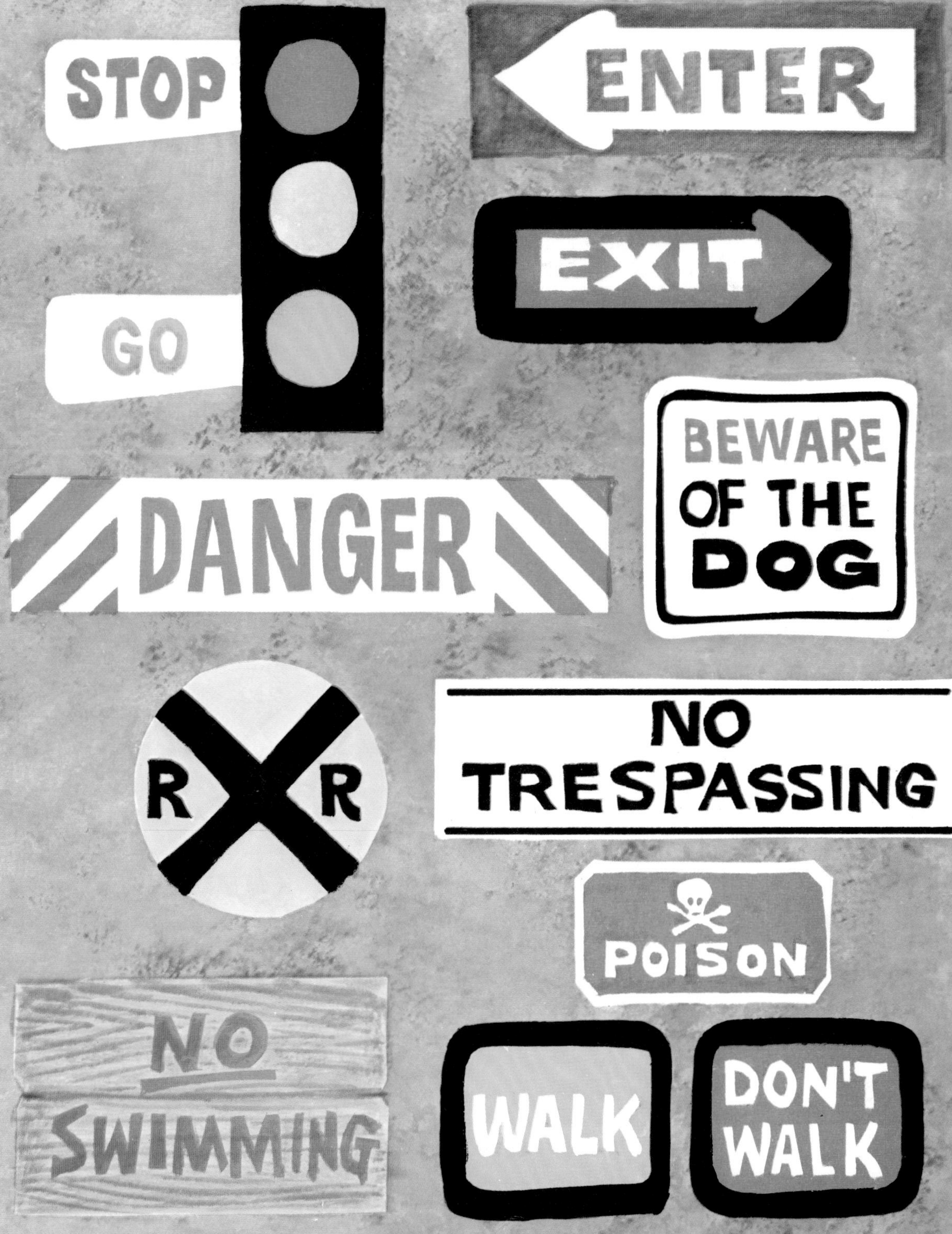

STOP

GO

ENTER

EXIT

DANGER

BEWARE
OF THE
DOG

R R

NO
TRESPASSING

POISON

NO
SWIMMING

WALK

DON'T
WALK

About the Author: Virginia Maniglier-Poulet lives with her husband and two young children in Tulsa, Oklahoma. After graduating as a fashion design major from Washington University in St. Louis, she designed women's lingerie for a year, then served in the Peace Corps in Morocco for two years. Recognizing a definite need for very simple, yet stimulating beginning readers, she developed her first book, *Blue Bug and the Bullies.* She feels that the illustration should catch the child's interest and stimulate him to try to actually READ the WORD, not read the picture. Her children's criticisms were pertinent to the development of both *Blue Bug and the Bullies* and *Blue Bug's Safety Book.*

About the Artist; Donald Charles started his long career as an artist more than twenty-five years ago after attending the University of California & the Art League School of California. He began by writing and illustrating feature articles for the San Francisco Chronicle, and also sold cartoons and ideas to The New Yorker and Cosmopolitan magazines. Since then he has been, at various times, a longshoreman, ranch hand, truck driver, and editor of a weekly newspaper, all enriching experiences for an artist. Ultimately he became creative director for an advertising agency, a post which he resigned several years ago to devote himself full-time to book illustration and writing. Mr. Charles has received frequent awards from graphic societies, and his work has appeared in numerous textbooks and periodicals. He and his artist wife have restored a turn-of-the-century frame house in Chicago where they live with their three children.